18 Beauty Recipes

Greatest Beauty Secrets of All Time!

Ann Savage

ANTI-AGING SKINCARE SECRETS REVEALED

How to have your skin Beautiful In

The Next 10 Days

Your Free Gift

As a way of saying thanks for your purchase, I'm offering a free guide that's exclusive to my readers.

In this guide, you will learn how to turn any messy room in into a nice, clean, and tidy room, cleaning in only 3 hours. Your home will stay clean every day and you will never have to worry about unexpected guests walking into a dirty house again. You can download this free report by going here.

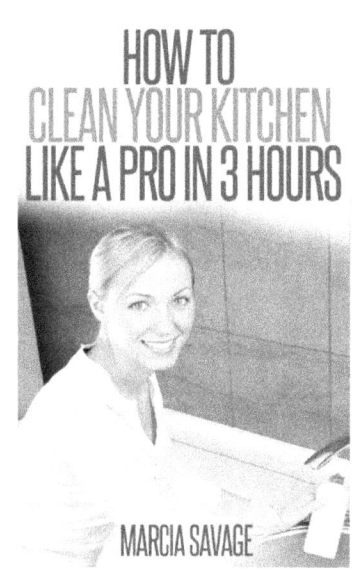

http://forms.aweber.com/form/76/315836976.htm

Table of Contents:

Who said you need a $10,000.00 face lift to look younger? During winter, summer, and fall, skin care is very important. Dry skin is the cause of wrinkles, and wrinkles can add 10 to 15 years on your face and hands. Well, surprise, surprise, and surprise, in this guide, you will find several homemade remedy to remove common body scars fast.

You don't need to be rich or have a rich uncle to take years off your appearance! Just try the beauty secrets inside the pages of this guide. You will be amazed with the results.

Hello! My name is Marcia Savage and thank you for purchasing my book. Inside this guide, I have put together sure-fire ingredients that will help you.

I know you're not a child but inside this book, I break the remedy down into a simple step by step formula anyone can follow. I'll show you the same ways it was shown to me by my mother and grandmother, skin care secrets handed down to them from their grandparents. These are people who could afford blackhead, acne remover treatment, or dental care but learned how to remove these common body scars and yellow stains from their teeth using home remedies.

So, get a pen and some paper and check out how you can cure almost any scar from your skin for 75% less than store brought treatments. Let's get started!

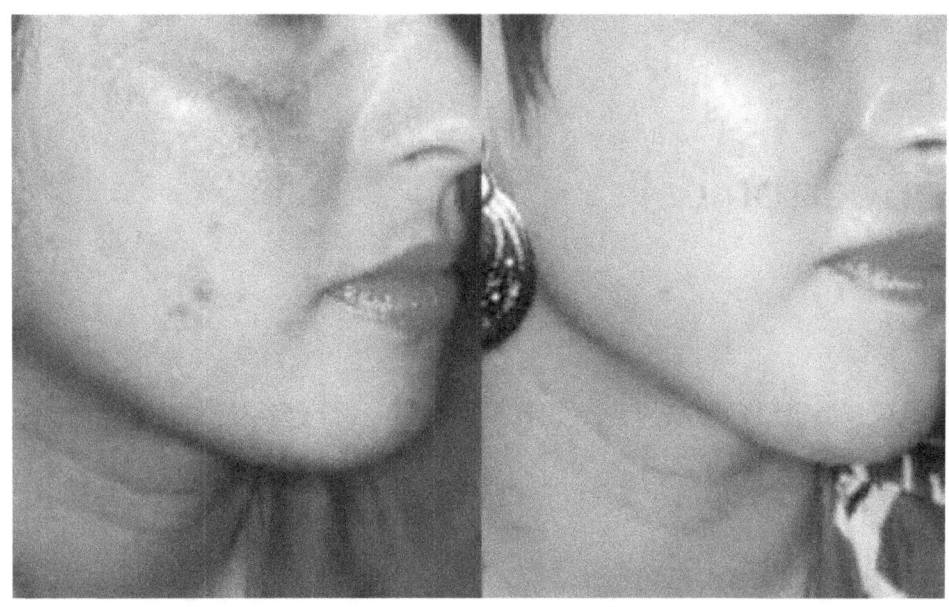

Do you want to get rid of acne without spending a ton of cash on expensive scar cream? Don't worry, I'm not trying to sell you another product. I'm sure you have tried them all. Here's my secret to help you get rid of acne scars fast.

You'll need:

Lemon

Q-Tip or Cotton balls

Step One: Squeeze ½ a lemon into your bowl. If you are worried about putting the pure lemon juice on your skin, add water.

Step Two: Dip a cotton ball into the lemon juice and swab it over the scar area.

Step Three: Leave it on for 30 minutes and rinse with warm water.

How To Make An Anti-Aging Banana Mask

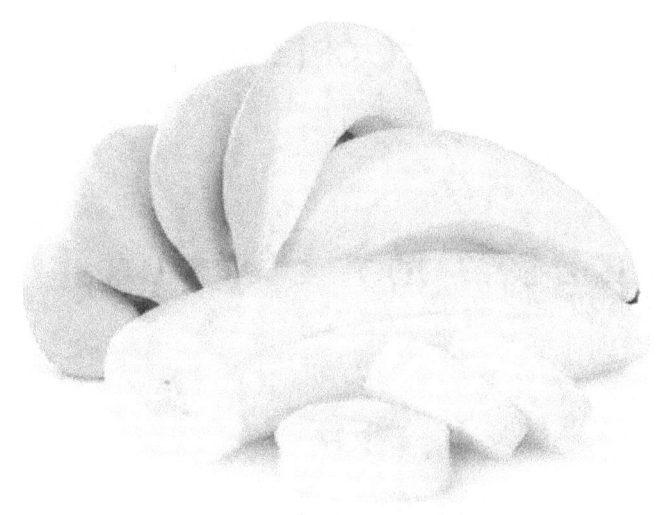

You'll need:

½ of a ripe banana

1 teaspoon honey

2 teaspoon honey

Step One: Mash ½ of a ripe banana into your bowl. Banana is great for your skin. A banana nourishes and rejuvenates skin with the essential nutritive elements like potassium, calcium, and vitamin C.

Step Two: Pour 2 teaspoon of yogurt in your bowl.

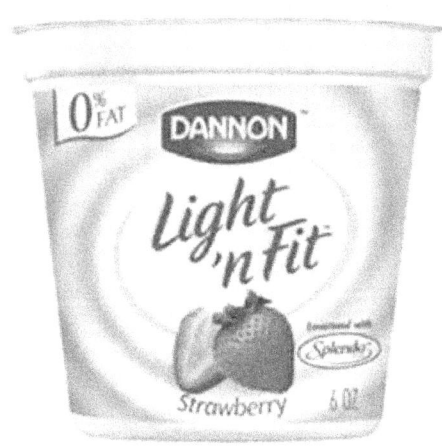

I get Dannon from Kroger's but any

yogurt will work!

Step Three: Pour in 2 teaspoons of honey and mix the solution well.

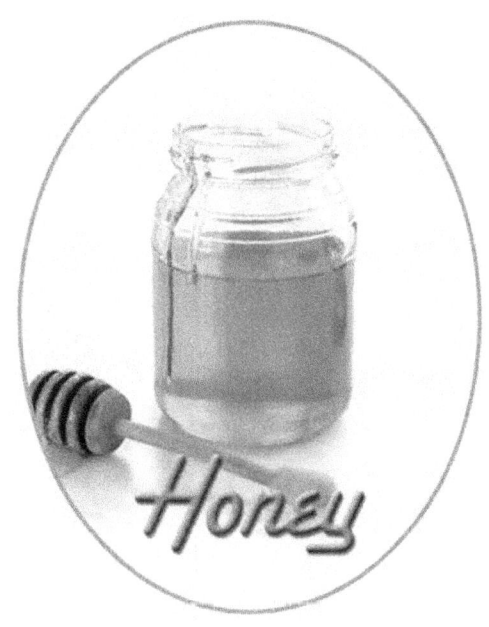

Honey is good for skin because it's a natural moisturizer and should be added to your skin care regimen.

Step Three: Apply the solution to your face and keep on for 20 minutes. Rinse your face with warm water.

How To Make A Banana Cream Mask

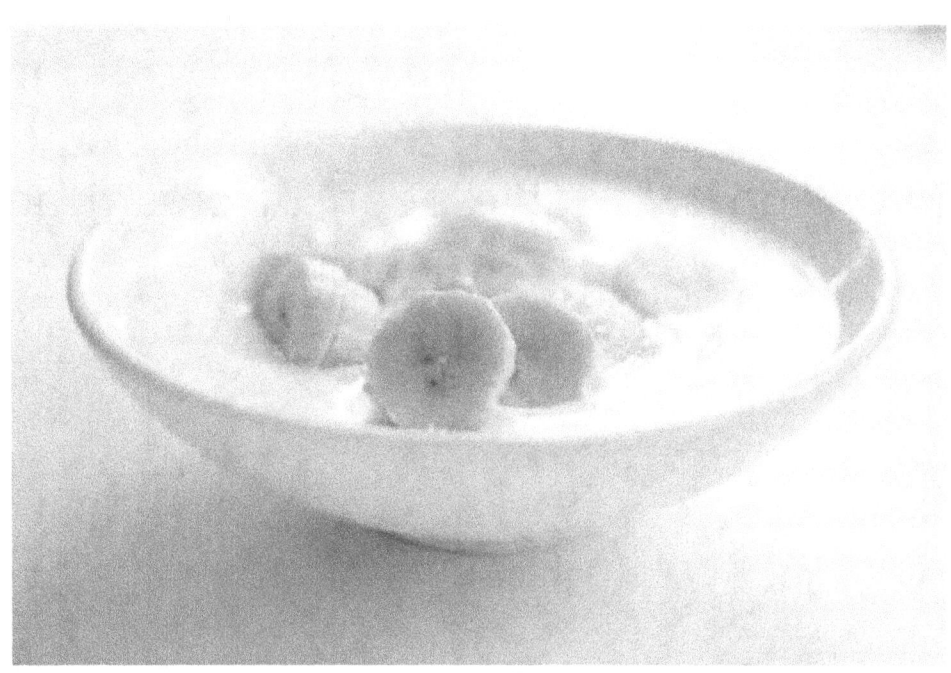

You'll need:

Potato flour

Cream

1 ripe Banana

Step One: Mash your banana in a bowl into a paste.

Step Two: Add two tablespoon of cream and mix well.

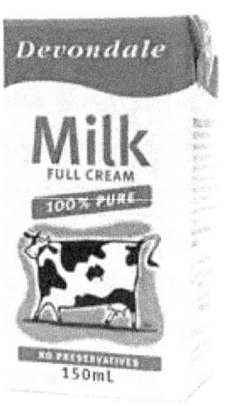

This is the milk cream I use. You can find it at Wal-Mart and it works best for dry skin. But any cream milk will do, check your dairy department.

Did you know that Cleopatra was known for taking milk baths? It was the secret to her naturally glowing skin.

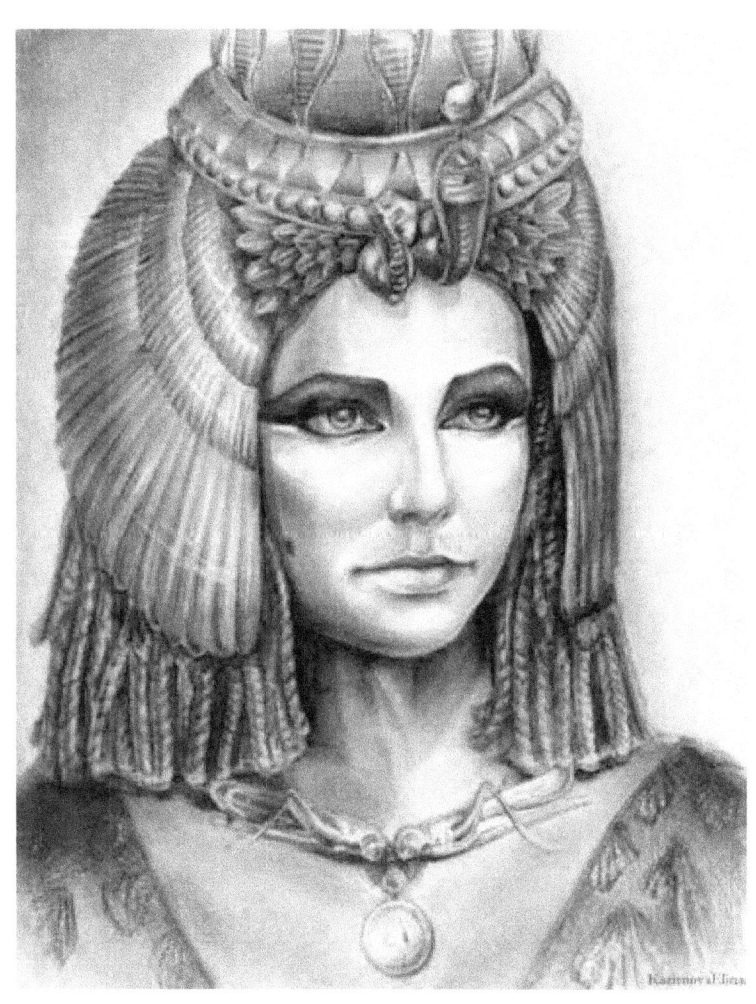

Step Three: Add one tablespoon of potato flour to the bowl and mix. Add enough flour and keep mixing until the solution becomes very dense. You can purchase potato flour at any of the follow sites.

http://www.nextag.com/Potato-Flour-Where-To-Buy/products-html?nxtg=19e10a3c051a-1BB8D026712442AB

http://www.pricemachine.com/Potato-Flour-Where-To-Buy/products-html?nxtg=169c0a50051a-E22DDDB91CAE6DCC

http://www.amazon.com/Sweet-Potato-Flour-1-lb/dp/B000FA6GY4

Step Four: Apply the first layer to your skin and let dry. Then apply the second layer.

Step Five: Leave the solution on for 30 minutes, and wash with warm water.

How To Make Homemade Wrinkle Cream

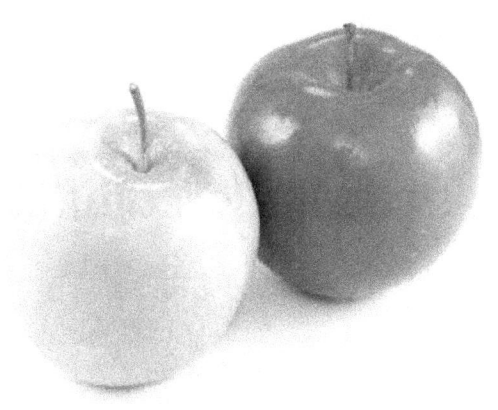

You need:

¼ of an apple

½ cup Soy milk

Blender

Hot Water

1 large Bowl & 1 small bowl

Cloth

Step One: Cut apple in half and blend into a paste.

Put the apple into the small bowl, pour ½ cup of hot water into the large bowl and set the small bowl inside the large bowl on top of the water.

Step Three: Pour ½ cup of soy Milk over the apple paste and mix slowly. Let the solution set for 5 minutes. This will give the vitamin A in the apple time to mix with the vitamin D in the milk.

Step Four: After five minutes, dip the cloth into the solution and apply to your skin. Leave on your skin for 20 minutes and rinse with warm water.

.

How To Get Rid Of Blackheads

You'll need:

Toothpaste

1 tablespoon Salt

Spoon

2 wash cloths

Step One: Pour enough toothpaste in the bowl to cover your face. Add one tablespoon of salt and mix.

Step Two: With the spoon, spread the mixture all over your face and leave it on for five minutes. Use caution around your eyes because if this mixture gets into your eye, it will burn.

Step Three: After five minutes, wet your cloth in warm water and lightly scrub your face.

Step Four: Wash off the mixture with cold water to complete the treatment.

If you have dry skin, use this skin treatment once a week. If you don't have dry skin, it is safe to use it three times a week.

How To Get Rid Of Whiteheads

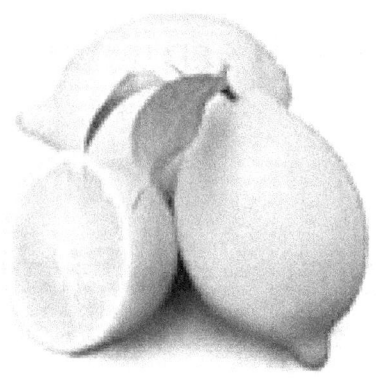

You'll need:

Clean Cloth

Lemon Juice

Water

Sugar

Cotton Balls

Step One: Wet your face with warm water.

Step Two: Take a cotton ball and soak it with lemon juice.

Step Three: Pour a teaspoon of sugar on the cotton ball.

Step Four: Take your cotton ball and lightly scrub your face. Give a lot of attention to the infected area.

Step Five: Rinse your face with warm water. This solution is safe to use three times a week. If your skin is sensitive to the lemon juice, dilute with water.

You'll need:

3 Eggs

Step One: Crack the eggs over a bowl, separate the white from the yolk and put the white in the bowl. Throw the yolk of the egg away.

Step Two: Massage the egg whites gently on your face and leave on for 30 minutes.

Step Three: Wash off the eggs with warm water and repeat this process three times a week. You'll be amazed at the results.

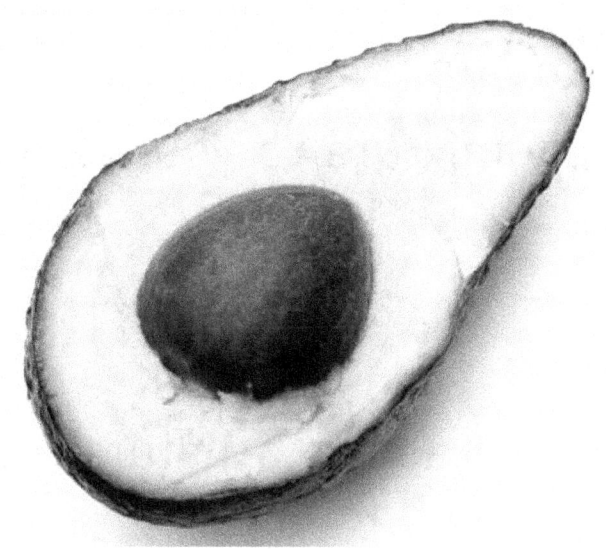

You'll need:

½ Avocados

2 tbsp. of cream

2 tsp. of flaxseeds

1 tbsp. of honey

Step One: Mash the avocado into a paste, add the other items into the bowl, and mix well.

Step Two: Apply mixture to your skin and leave on for 2 hours.

Did you know avocado is a natural moisturizer for dry skin?

Step Three: Wash the mixture off with warm water and pat dry with a towel.

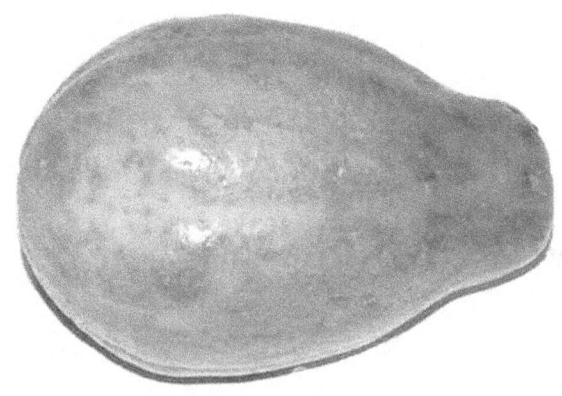

You'll need:

¼ Papayas

1 ripe banana

Bowl

Step One: Mash the papaya and banana into a paste inside the bowl.

Step Two: Apply mixture to skin and leave on for 30 minutes.

Step Three: Wash off with warm water and repeat this process twice a week.

You'll need:

4 tbsp. of wheat flour

½ tsp. Turmeric powder

1 tsp. Mustard Oil

Step One: Pour all ingredients into a bowl, slowly add warm water and mix into a paste.

Step Two: Apply mixture to your skin and allow it to dry.

Step Three: Once it's dry, remove by scrubbing it off with a clean cloth.

Step Four: Leave the film on your skin for 20 minutes and wash off with warm water.

Repeat this process four times a week for dry skin.

You need:

2 tbsp. Honey

2 tsp. Milk

Step One: Pour the milk and honey into a bowl and mix into a paste.

Step Two: Apply mixture on your skin and leave it on for 30 minutes.

Step Three: After 30 minutes, wash off with warm water.

Repeat this process three times a week for dry skin.

In the warm seasons, you should moisturize your skin once a day. In the winter, you should moisturize your skin twice a day. This will keep your skin looking 10 years younger throughout your life.

You need:

Olive Oil

Warm water

Clean Cloth

Step One: Wash your skin in warm water. Keeping your skin clean keeps it moisturizer.

Don't wash your skin in hot water because hot water strips the oils from your, causing dry and wrinkled skin.

Step Two: Apply olive oil over your skin, completely covering the dry areas.

Cover your skin with a warm, dry cloth and keep it on until the cloth is cool.

Step Three: Wipe the solution off your skin and wash with warm water.

Make this part of your skin care regimen after daily baths.

You'll need:

2 tbsp. Olive Oil

½ Cup Sugar

Step One: Mix the solution into a paste.

Step Two: Apply the solution to your skin and leave it on for 5 minutes.

Step Three: Wash it off with warm water.

You'll need:

2 tbsp. of Plain Yogurt

1 tbsp. of grated Almonds

1 Egg York

Step One: Pour these ingredients in a bowl and mix into a paste.

Step Two: Apply the solution to your face and leave it on for 5 minutes.

Step Three: Wash away with warm water.

You'll need:

1 ripe Banana

1 tbsp. of Olive Oil

Step One: Mash the banana into a paste and mix with the Olive Oil in your bowl.

Step Two: Apply it to your face and leave on for 15 minutes.

Step Three: Wash off the solution with warm water.

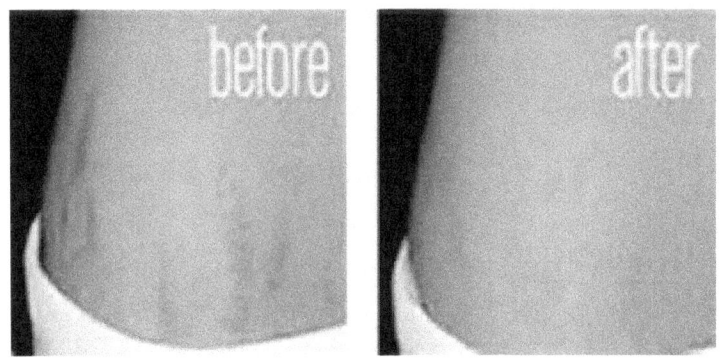

You'll need:

1 tbsp. Sugar

2 tbsp. Almond Oil

Step One: Pour the solution into a bowl and mix well.

Step Two: Rub the mixture into the scarred area for five minutes.

Step Three: Repeat this process twice a week until the scars disappear.

This solution will stimulate collagen through exfoliation to remove stretch marks.

How To Have Whiter Teeth In 3 Minutes

You'll need:

1 tsp. Baking Soda

½ Orange

Step One: Pour the baking soda into a bowl and squeeze the juice from the orange on the soda.

Step Two: Mix the solution well and let set for 5 minutes until it stops foaming.

Step Four: Apply the solution on your teeth with your finger and keep it on 4 minutes.

Step Five: Rinse your mouth a warm water.

For best results, repeat this process three times a week.

.

You'll need:

Baking Soda

Tooth Brush

Warm Water

Step One: Rinse your mouth several times with water.

Step Two: Pour 1 tablespoon of baking soda in a clean bowl. Add ¼ cup of warm water and mix into a paste.

Step Three: Take you tooth brush dip it in the mixture and brush your teeth for two minutes.

Step Four: Rinse your mouth until the mixture gone.

If you want whiter teeth, repeat this process 3 times a day.

Four Proven Ways To Whiten
Extremely Yellow Teeth

Number One:

You'll need:

Strawberries

Baking Soda

Step One: Take two strawberries and mash them up in a bowl add one teaspoon of baking soda and mix to a paste.

Step Two: Put the mixture on a brush and brush your teeth for one minute.

One Three: Rinse your mouth with warm water.

Number Two:

You'll need

1 tsp. Baking Soda

1 tsp. White Vinegar

This mixture foams I wouldn't mix it in a bowl that is too small for the chemical reaction.

Step One: Pour the ingredients in a bowl and mix into a paste.

Step Two: Put the mixture on a tooth brush and brush your teeth for two minutes.

Step Three: Rinse your mouth several times with warm water.

Number Three

You'll need:

1 tbsp. Olive Oil

Cotton Balls

Step One: Pour one tablespoon of Olive Oil in a bowl and dip the cotton ball in the olive oil.

Step Two: Run the cotton ball over your teeth.

Repeat this process daily for two weeks for best results.

Thank you so much for taking the time to read this book. I hope your skin care regimen is an easy and simple process.

Now I'd like ask for a *small* favor. If you found this book to be useful, please take a few minutes to leave a review on Amazon...

...Even a few sentences will help!

Here's the link again:

amazon.com/author/marciasavage e

This feedback will help me to write the kind of Kindle books that help you get results. And if you loved it, please let me know.

More Kindle eBooks By Marcia Savage:

CLEAN HOUSE IN 30 MINUTES

http://www.amazon.com/CLEAN-HOUSE-IN-30-MINUTES-ebook/dp/B00HVS4TZG

AN ORGANIZED HOME IN 30 MINUTES

http://www.amazon.com/AN-ORGANIZED-HOME-IN-MINUTES-ebook/dp/B00IGKZU0G

BEST HOMEMADE STAIN REMOVER EVER

http://www.amazon.com/BEST-HOMEMADE-STAIN-REMOVER-EVER-ebook/dp/B00IPQ1VF4

Kindle eBooks By Bernard Savage

At Last a Proven Way to Housebreak Your Dog

http://www.amazon.com/Last-Proven-Way-Housebreak-Your-ebook/dp/B00GS174JK

At Last, a Proven Way to Train a Well-Behaved Dog

http://www.amazon.com/dp/B00GWBEUYS

The Easy Way to Housebreak Your Dog in 10 Days

http://www.amazon.com/The-Easy-Housebreak-Your-Days-ebook/dp/B00HK9BIGE

The Easy Way to Teach Your Dog to Come In 10 Days

http://www.amazon.com/EASY-TEACH-YOUR-COME-DAYS-ebook/dp/B00HL24R40

The Easy Way to Train a Well-Behaved Dog in 10 Days

http://www.amazon.com/The-Easy-Train-Well-Behaved-Days-ebook/dp/B00HKUTB3A

GUARATTEE PROVEN RESULTS! TEACH YOUR DOG TO COME WHEN YOU CALL IN 10 DAYS

http://www.amazon.com/dp/B00H5CE3Y0

The Absolute Quickest Way to start a Window Cleaning Business

http://www.amazon.com/Absolute-Quickest-Window-Cleaning-Business-ebook/dp/B00GIS2LZA

The Absolute Cheapest Way to start a Doggy Daycare Business

http://www.amazon.com/dp/B00GKPDWFO

The Fastest Way to Start a Successful Pet Grooming Business

http://www.amazon.com/dp/B00GISLRQY

The Fast Way to start a Car Detailing Business

http://www.amazon.com/Fast-Way-start-Detailing-Business-ebook/dp/B00GH565ME